Litigation Assistant

A GUIDE FOR THE DEFENDANT PHYSICIAN

Second Edition

Litigation Assistant

A GUIDE FOR THE DEFENDANT PHYSICIAN

Second Edition

*This publication has been made possible
by a grant from the Committee on
Development of the American College
of Obstetricians and Gynecologists*

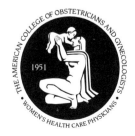

Department of Professional Liability
American College of Obstetricians and Gynecologists

Litigation Assistant: A Guide for the Defendant Physician, Second Edition, was developed by the staff of the Department of Professional Liability of the American College of Obstetricians and Gynecologists.

Department of Professional Liability Staff:
Larry P. Griffin, MD, FACOG, Director, Program Services
Kenneth V. Heland, JD, Associate Director, Professional Liability
Susannah Jones, JD
Linda Esser
Charlene Burger

ISBN 0-915473-45-3

Library of Congress Cataloging-in-Publication Data

Litigation assistant: a guide for the defendant physician /
    Department of Professional Liability, American College of Obstetricians and
    Gynecologists.—2nd Edition
        p.   cm.
    "This publication has been made possible by a grant from the Committee on
Development of the American College of Obstetricians and Gynecologists."
    Includes bibliographical references and index.
    ISBN 0-915473-45-3
    1. Obstetricians—Malpractice—United States—Trial practice. 2. Gynecologists—
Malpractice—United States—Trial practice. 3. Trial practice—United States.
    I. American College of Obstetricians and Gynecologists. Dept. of Professional
    Liability.
KF8925.M3L56   1998
344.73'04121—dc21   98-14138
                                                                            CIP

12345/21098

Contents

Dedication

This monograph is dedicated to Keith White, MD, FACOG, former director of ACOG and a major force behind better information for Fellows regarding risk management and professional liability issues. Dr. White's leadership, commitment, and diligent efforts on behalf of ACOG Fellows and Junior Fellows are evident in many areas of ACOG activities, but none more so than in the professional liability arena. It is with a great sense of pride and indebtedness that this edition of the *Litigation Assistant* is dedicated to him.

Preface

"Dear Doctor,

I represent a former patient of yours who suffers as a result of your negligent diagnosis and treatment. Please forward a complete copy of her medical records to my office. Enclosed is a signed release for this information. Thank you for your prompt attention in this matter.

Sincerely,"

We hope you never receive a letter like this one, but, unfortunately, especially as obstetricians and gynecologists, lawsuits are an all-too-common occurrence. We know that nothing can prevent the possibility of a claim of negligence being made against you. We also know that once that claim is made, no matter how groundless it may be, a series of events begins that puts physicians in a strange world with different rules and procedures than any of us have dealt with in all the years of our education and training.

This monograph is intended to assist you in the event you become a participant in the medical–legal process. Various sections deal with the different phases or aspects of a professional liability lawsuit. The information is designed to help you understand the process and better prepare for your role in it. It is not intended to be a comprehensive course of preparation for the legal system. Instead, this monograph should be viewed as a primer to enable you to understand the process better and improve communication with your attorney. We also believe that, in addition to improving the ability of you and your attorney to work together, better understanding of the process and preparation on your part can improve your ability to deal with the situation both professionally and emotionally.

Each section can be read alone if you need information about a specific subject. We encourage you, however, to read the entire booklet, preferably at a time when you can do so without the pressure of impending litigation.

The information is intended to be helpful to you in your daily practice as you increase your awareness of ways to reduce your risk of liability exposure.

We hope you never have occasion to use this booklet in preparation for trial. In case you do, however, we hope you find it useful.

Larry P. Griffin, MD, FACOG
Director
Program Services

Litigation Assistant

A GUIDE FOR THE DEFENDANT PHYSICIAN

Second Edition

Introduction

The American College of Obstetricians and Gynecologists published the first edition of *Litigation Assistant: A Guide for the Defendant Physician* in 1986 to provide ACOG Fellows with the tools and skills to become better, more informed defendants in medical liability cases. The first edition of *Litigation Assistant* introduced the term *legal risk management* to the medical liability lexicon.

Unfortunately, legal risk management considerations still apply today. It is a virtual certainty that you will be subjected to a lawsuit at least once during your career. Seventy-three percent of ACOG members have been sued at least once. The typical obstetrician–gynecologist experiences 2.3 lawsuits during the first 14 years of medical practice. Lawsuits are still a fact of life for the practicing ob-gyn.

The American College of Obstetricians and Gynecologists has worked extensively for reform of the medical malpractice system, both at the state and federal level. Some of that reform has involved creative alternatives to the current tort system, such as the birth-related neurologic injury compensation funds in Virginia and Florida. Until additional reforms of that nature come about, ob-gyns must deal with the realities of the present system. Members of ACOG still need to know how to practice legal risk management in the event that they are sued.

The Department of Professional Liability has regular contact with ACOG members who are in the midst of the litigation process. In many instances, this is the member's first exposure to the U.S. judicial system. It is an unpleasant and traumatic experience, to say the least. However, the College feels that information of the nature contained in the *Litigation Assistant* can help.

An informed defendant is one who understands the process and is aware of his or her rights and responsibilities with respect to the other participants. Although we recognize and empathize with the natural tendency on the part of ACOG members to avoid the process because of the trauma, a truly informed and strong defendant can help improve the outcome of the litigation.

The *Litigation Assistant* has separate sections dealing with each element of the lawsuit process in the sequence in which they occur. Each section is written with a principal focus on the defendant physician. There is no need to read the entire book in order; for example, if you currently are involved in litigation and have an upcoming Deposition, you may want to read that section first. You should specifically read the section on professional liability insurance and incident management, regardless of whether you currently are involved in litigation. Much has changed in the insurance field since the publication of the first edition.

The National Practitioner Data Bank was implemented after the original publication of *Litigation Assistant*. Reports to the Data Bank of medical liability settlements may have an impact on your future insurability, your clinical privileges and institutions, and your managed care contracts.

The appendix contains three sections that may be of interest as well. The "Commonsense Glossary of Medical–Legal Terms" defines and explains terms that arise in the text and the lawsuit process. The "Cross-Reference Index of Medical–Legal Terms" groups terms into lists by subject, such as professional liability insurance, settlement, and trial. And for those of you who wish to review this subject more extensively, "Suggested Reading" points the way to some of the best and most comprehensive books in the field.

The information in this publication should not be construed as legal advice. This book is not intended to supplant or replace your attorney's advice. The Department of Professional Liability is available as a reference to you during litigation, and you should feel free to contact the department at any time with questions.

Our closing to the introduction to the first edition still applies today: It is our hope that you will save this book in your library and readily consult it as needed. It is our personal wish that you may never need to consult it. It is our desire and goal that the ultimate reform of the system may make much of this book obsolete. Until then, may you be comforted by the fact that it is available.

Professional
Liability Insurance

Purchasing professional liability insurance is one of the most important and most expensive decisions you will ever make. Thoughtful consideration and examination should be made before the purchase of this insurance. It is essential to know the exact type of policy being bought, as well as the reputation, history, and financial stability of the insurance carrier. It is always a good idea to check with your state insurance department for information about the carrier. However, there are some insurance programs, such as risk-retention groups and self-insurance funds, that are not necessarily required to register in all states where they do business. Your state's insurance insolvency fund will not provide protection for unregistered insurance companies. A risk-retention group is required only to register with the insurance department in its state of incorporation. Self-insurance funds may not have to register at all.

In today's insurance market, you need to consider both availability and affordability of professional liability insurance. With the emergence of risk-retention groups and self-insurance funds, you have more of a choice regarding insurance carrier or type of policy. As a result, insurance premiums have become more competitive.

As a part of your investigation, you should attempt to obtain a sample copy of the policy and read the contents. A cheaper premium is not always a better buy. It is a good idea to have your personal attorney review the sample policy. You should also inquire about the insurance company's underwriting criteria for termination, cancellation, nonrenewal, and surcharges. Consider how those criteria would affect your practice. Determine whether the policy allows the insurance entity to collect additional premiums from you at a later date if its losses are high and its reserves are inadequate.

As in any relationship or contract, each party to the insurance policy has responsibilities and obligations to the other. The insurance company agrees to accept financial responsibility on behalf of the insured for payment of any judgment or settlement, up to a specific monetary limit, in return for a fee (premium). In addition, the company is usually financially responsible

3

for investigating a claim, negotiating a settlement, and defending the insured physician. In recent years, some insurance carriers have sought to limit these obligations with per-claim deductibles and limitations on defense costs. If your policy contains any of these special provisions, make sure that you fully understand them and how they would apply to your practice.

You must know what is stated in your professional liability policies and what requirements and obligations are placed upon you. You will usually be required to notify your carriers as soon as a claim is made or suspected. A fear exists among many physicians that their premiums will increase or that their policies will be canceled as a result of early notification of an incident or claim. Although this might be a legitimate concern in some instances, your insurance company may be able to deny coverage of a claim that is not promptly reported. However, there are advantages to early notification. Early notification aids in early evaluation and preparation of a case, which, in turn, improves the chances of a successful defense should an actual claim develop. Such action affords the insurance company the opportunity to begin collecting and recording facts early and evaluating the case for merit. In some instances, it may be able to negotiate an early settlement with the claimant before litigation begins. You should be aware that payments, including settlements, made on your behalf in a medical malpractice case are required to be reported to the National Practitioner Data Bank. However, individual physicians are no longer required to report payments they make on their own behalf. Also, an important factor to keep in mind is that any written or recorded information given to your insurance company is not privileged and is subject to discovery by the plaintiff. Therefore, you should direct all communication related to the claim to your defense attorney once one has been assigned to your case, because information given to your attorney is protected by the attorney–client privilege and is not discoverable.

You have a duty to cooperate with your insurance companies in the defense of your cases, and failure to do so could cause the policy to be voided. Therefore, to meet the obligation to cooperate with your assigned defense attorney, you must candidly and in good faith discuss all aspects of the case so that there are no surprises.

Some insurance companies require claims to be reviewed by a committee of physicians, often in the relevant specialty, before a decision is made to defend or settle a claim. An insurance company may, by the terms of the policy, have the right to settle a claim without your consent, but you should try to involve yourself in this decision as much as possible. You might be able to use the National Practitioner Data Bank reporting requirement to involve yourself in settlement discussions.

You also may have personal reasons why settlement is worth consideration. Expense, time loss, and mental and emotional strain are always associated with litigation. You may realize that there is more at risk, both financially and professionally, than initially anticipated and believe that settlement is the best option. All these issues should be discussed thoroughly with your insurance carrier and defense attorney before arriving at a decision to make a settlement offer. In addition, your insurance carrier may have a litigation support group program that can help you cope with litigation stress and help you make clear, focused decisions about the course of the litigation. If your defense counsel recommends settling, ask for an explanation justifying a settlement. A good rapport among you, your carrier, and your defense attorney will aid in achieving such requests.

Another major concern for you may be the possible need for personal defense counsel. The typical professional liability policy gives the insurer the right to select counsel and control the defense of a claim. However, there may be instances when personal defense counsel is warranted. Your insurance company is only obligated to pay an award up to the liability limits of your policy. If the potential verdict in your case exceeds the liability limits of your policy, your insurer should let you know and should advise you of your right to obtain personal defense counsel at your own expense. Keep in mind that if you hire your own defense attorney, the insurance company's defense attorney will continue to defend your claim at the company's expense.

A problem that may arise is one of coverage. Your insurance carrier may question whether you were insured for a particular procedure or whether your policy was in effect at the time of the incident. In such circumstances, your carrier customarily will send you a "reservation of rights" letter in which it will agree to defend you but will reserve the right to contest the coverage problem until after the malpractice case is resolved. With the increasing popularity of "gyn-only" policies and the use of exclusions to limit coverage for certain treatments or procedures, this issue could become increasingly significant. Engaging in procedures that go beyond the scope of your covered practice will create problems. When you receive a reservation of rights letter, you are strongly advised to retain your own personal defense counsel. In addition, if at any time during the litigation process you feel that your best interests are not being protected, you have the right to obtain your own personal defense attorney.

It is vital to keep the actual insurance policy after it has expired. With the growth in mergers and acquisitions of insurance companies, you should not assume that the insurance company will keep a record of your policy on file. You may be required to prove that you were insured for an incident, and the policy itself is the best evidence.

Incident Management

An incident is an event that suggests the possibility of a medical malpractice lawsuit. Your appropriate management of an incident is of the utmost importance. A delay in reporting a suspected problem could make it difficult to prepare a successful defense.

Your first reactions to an incident can be critical to the outcome of a potential or actual lawsuit. You need to know what is stated in your professional liability policy and what requirements and obligations are placed upon you. Usually you will be required to notify your carrier as soon as a claim is made or suspected. Physicians often are afraid that their premiums will increase or that their policies will be canceled as a result of early notification of an incident or claim. Although there may be a legitimate concern in some instances, early notification aids in early evaluation and preparation of a case, which, in turn, improves the chances of a successful defense should an actual claim develop. Such action affords the insurance company the opportunity to begin collecting and recording facts early and evaluating the case for merit.

SIGNS OF A POTENTIAL LAWSUIT

The most obvious scenario indicating the potential for a lawsuit is an unexpected outcome or complication during the treatment of your patient. You might receive direct complaints or expressions of dissatisfaction with an outcome from the patient or the patient's family. Another sign is being contacted by an attorney requesting information on a patient's treatment. A request for medical records might be made by an attorney, another physician, or the patient herself. Remember that a request might be written or verbal. You must have written authorization from the patient before you release any information. You should send copies of the requested records and retain the originals for your files. You might want to keep a list of all records that have been provided and to whom.

There are more subtle indications that a patient may be dissatisfied and, therefore, prone to filing a lawsuit. You should be cautious with your noncompliant patients. If a patient refuses a medical test/procedure, or even hospitalization, you should note your informed consent discussions with that patient in that patient's file. In such cases, you may even want the patient to sign a form indicating her refusal for the specific treatment.

If a patient fails to keep scheduled follow-up visits, you should document your efforts to contact her. Also, a patient who fails to pay or unnecessarily delays payment of a bill could be dissatisfied and contemplating a lawsuit. You might assuage such patients with personal inquiries reflecting your concern with their satisfaction and possibly offer to establish a payment schedule if that would assist them.

RESPONDING TO AN INCIDENT

Sometimes the simplest of acts in response to an incident can help avoid a lawsuit. If your patient has experienced an unexpected bad outcome, some experts recommend that you honestly explain what happened to the patient and her family and express empathy. If appropriate, this is an opportunity for you to offer further medical or surgical procedures to help alleviate the situation. Above all, don't avoid contact with the patient or her family at this stage. You would not want to be perceived as having something to hide.

You should put your insurance carrier on notice about an unexpected outcome. Again, this will give you a head start in the event of litigation. If you have a claims-made policy, only claims that are reported during the policy period will be covered. If the event occurred at the hospital, you need to notify the risk manager or incident manager there.

You might find it helpful to review your patient's medical record. You will want to be familiar with the details of the specific case.

An important factor to keep in mind is that any written or recorded information given to your insurance company is not privileged and is subject to discovery. Therefore, you should direct all communication related to the claim to your defense attorney once one has been assigned to your case, because information given to your attorney is protected by the attorney–client privilege.

If a formal claim has been filed, you should not attempt to negotiate directly with the patient or her attorney because it could harm your defense should a lawsuit follow. If you do have contact with the patient or her family concerning the incident, you should make contemporaneous written notes of all oral communications. Also, any correspondence you may have regarding the incident should be saved in a separate file from the patient's medical records.

Claims Management

A lawsuit begins when the plaintiff files a formal Complaint or Declaration, a legal document consisting of allegations, the legal basis to support a claim for medical malpractice against the defendant, and a request for damages or other relief. Once a Complaint or Declaration has been filed, the court serves each defendant with a Summons. The Summons usually is attached to the Complaint or Declaration and requires the defendant to file a response, usually known as an Answer, within a specified period of time.

Your defense attorney will prepare the Answer and must respond to each of the allegations and issues. Failure to file an Answer may result in a default judgment against you. Failure to respond to allegations or issues may be considered an admission of culpability. *This matter deserves immediate attention: Answers must be filed quickly (usually within 30 days from the date you receive the Summons), and there are stringent penalties for not responding.*

RESPONDING TO A FORMAL CLAIM

You should notify your professional liability insurance company immediately so that you and your attorney can respond appropriately to the Complaint or Declaration. Your insurance company usually will tell you the name of the attorney and the law firm assigned to your defense immediately after the lawsuit has been filed, if not before. With you as a resource person, your attorney will prepare a written Answer to be filed within the time prescribed by the Summons. Your attorney must respond to each allegation and issue contained in the Complaint or Declaration.

You should deliver the Summons (including the attached Complaint or Declaration) to your defense attorney and/or your insurance carrier. A photocopy should be retained for your records.

You may wish to prepare a thorough analysis of the case for your attorney. This could include a detailed, complete evaluation of all medical files, such as all records, correspondence, X-rays, and lab tests. If requested by your defense attorney, you should prepare a chronologic documentation of the medical data, including everything you know about your case and treatment of the patient. Materials that you prepare at the request of your attorney in preparation for litigation are not subject to discovery by the plaintiff's counsel because they are considered attorney work product. You should keep all of this information in a file separate from the patient's records.

You must not alter the medical records in any way. Evidence of tampering with the records can lead to a loss of credibility in court as well as a substantial increase in the size of an award. Most legal commentators agree that tampered records render a case indefensible. Sophisticated scientific techniques are now available to prove alterations or tampering.

You should never send originals of requested records, only photocopies. Before you release any information, you should check with your attorney and be certain to have proper authorization from your patient.

You might offer to serve as a medical educational resource for your defense team. In this role, you can review textbooks and medical articles relating to the medical issues in the case and conduct MEDLINE searches, if possible. You can educate your defense team about the strengths and weaknesses of the medical aspects of your case. It is important that your attorneys know about differing viewpoints and alternative treatments.

Your relationship with your insurance representative and your attorney needs to be honest, open, and truthful. Any unanticipated facts will come as a surprise, which is the worst nightmare of a defense attorney.

Above all, you should stay calm. Your first reactions to a Summons may be surprise, anger, panic, and self-doubt. It is unproductive to overreact or be hostile. There is much to do, and being levelheaded is essential in preparing a successful defense.

Working with Your Defense Attorney

It is important to meet with your defense attorney as soon as possible after the lawsuit begins. When you get the information from your insurance company about the attorney assigned to your case, you should call to arrange an appointment. It is vital to the outcome of your case that you feel comfortable and have good rapport with your defense attorney.

Your first meeting can be considered an evaluation period. If you encounter any problems with this relationship that cannot be directly resolved with your attorney, you should discuss your concerns with your insurance company. Most insurance carriers will be very attentive to your problems and try to resolve them, because a good attorney–client relationship is essential to a successful defense. Never be afraid to ask questions of your attorney or insurance company if you have any concerns.

EVALUATING YOUR ATTORNEY

Your primary objective of the evaluation of your attorney is to determine whether he or she is the best person to handle the defense of your lawsuit. Although this determination is often subjective, there are some considerations to keep in mind. Does your attorney understand the medicine involved in your case? If not, is your attorney willing and motivated to learn the medicine? Does your attorney have experience handling similar types of medical malpractice claims? What is the reputation of your attorney and of his or her law firm? Is your attorney well regarded by other legal colleagues and the community as a whole? Your personal attorney for your family or medical practice can help with this evaluation.

The most prestigious and highly regarded attorney will not be of much help in your defense if he or she is consumed with other legal matters. You should be concerned if your attorney seems too busy or does not have time for you. Canceled appointments, unreturned phone calls, or frequent interruptions during pretrial preparation meetings can be a manifestation of this problem.

You should be aware that the defense of medical malpractice claims is a team effort by many law firms. Even in such circumstances, however, you should determine the extent of involvement of your lead defense counsel. For example, will your lead counsel personally handle your deposition and that of the opposing expert witnesses and the plaintiff? Will your lead counsel be the primary attorney at the actual trial? What is the projected role of the law firm's associates and paralegals in handling your defense? Sometimes the insurance company has an agreement that specifies exact involvement of lead counsel in the defense of claims and minimizes the uncontrolled involvement of associates and paralegals. If you are having difficulty getting answers to these questions from your attorney, do not hesitate to contact your insurance company.

Personality can also play a role in building a successful attorney–client relationship. You do not have to be a close, personal friend of your attorney, but you should be able to communicate well and feel comfortable with each other.

Cases involving multiple defendants are common in obstetrics and gynecology malpractice cases. Insurance companies often suggest that the same attorney provide the defense for several defendants in the case, such as other physicians or the hospital. If you are presented with such a situation, you should be attuned to potential conflicts of interest. For example, there may be a factual dispute between you and the other codefendants. You should ask your attorney how this will be handled so that any potential arguments that could be raised on your behalf will not be sacrificed to the common defense.

It is often illuminating to discuss conflicts of interest with the defense attorney assigned by your insurance carrier, because this issue can give rise to other potential problems. Your attorney may demonstrate more allegiance to your insurance company than to you, especially if assigned malpractice litigation from your insurance company is a large portion of the law firm's business. You may be urged to forego retaining personal counsel in order to increase the strength of the common defense. This is a risky situation fraught with peril for you and your personal assets.

It is hoped that you will be satisfied with your defense attorney after you have completed this evaluation. At this point it is important for you and your attorney to begin to function as a defense team, which should increase the chances of a successful outcome to the lawsuit. You should be prepared to carry out your responsibilities to your attorney and understand your attorney's responsibilities to you.

RESPONSIBILITIES OF A DEFENDANT PHYSICIAN

Your primary responsibility as a defendant physician is to cooperate and participate in the defense of your case. It is helpful for you to learn how the legal process works in medical liability cases. Your attorney is an expert on litigation procedures, so listen to what he or she has to say about various stages of the process.

Medical liability litigation is a time-consuming process, especially in ob-gyn cases. You need to be prepared to set aside time from your schedule to work on your defense.

Even though you are the defendant physician, you should regard yourself as one of the medical experts for the defense team. You can offer to provide medical input to your attorney and discuss your role in preparing the medical defense. For example, you could research and provide medical literature relevant to the case and educate your attorney about the medical procedures involved in your lawsuit. You can help your attorney review and understand the medical records, and it is important to explain your treatment rationale. You can review the alternative treatments that you considered and rejected and help your attorney evaluate the medical strengths and weaknesses of your case.

Visual aids and exhibits can be helpful in educating the jury about the medicine involved; you should discuss this with your attorney and offer to provide assistance to your attorney in obtaining these exhibits. Also, because of the importance of expert witness testimony, you should offer to help your attorney identify noted experts in the field, especially those with special expertise on the condition or treatment involved in your case. You can also offer to help provide background information about the opposing medical experts. Finally, you can offer to help your attorney with jury selection—in smaller communities this is often helpful, because you may have background information on prospective jurors that your attorney does not have.

It is vital to maintain an open and honest dialogue with your attorney throughout the lawsuit process. If there is any information whatsoever that may be pertinent, you should disclose it to your attorney. Do not surprise your attorney with pertinent information at the last minute. You should regard yourself as your attorney's legal patient, and your attorney needs a complete history. Don't be shy or unduly deferential to your attorney; it is always better to ask questions and clear up any misunderstandings.

RESPONSIBILITIES OF YOUR DEFENSE ATTORNEY

Your attorney has many responsibilities to you during the course of the litigation. The proper fulfillment of these responsibilities will help to provide the best possible defense in your case.

Litigation is full of stress and anxiety for defendant physicians. Your attorney can help alleviate that stress somewhat by keeping you fully informed about the litigation process, explaining the significance of each stage of the proceedings, and thoroughly preparing you for your role in the process.

Your attorney must also carefully investigate the evidence and prepare the case by deciding on strategy and tactics. He or she must consider all of the factors that could win or lose your case, such as the status of the medical records, the severity of the injury, and the potential future damages for the plaintiff. Your attorney will also consider the appearance and credibility of the plaintiff and other plaintiff witnesses; your appearance and credibility, as well as that of your witnesses; and the quality and credibility of the expert witnesses for both sides. Other factors that must be considered and evaluated by your defense attorney include the ability and experience of the plaintiff's attorney and the trial judge assigned to the case, as well as any real or potential biases that the judge may have. The locale in which the case is to be tried (in particular, whether it is conservative or liberal in awarding damages), the caliber of the jurors, and the track record of similar cases previously settled or tried to a verdict in your jurisdiction are also important factors.

Frequent communication between you and your attorney is essential. It is important that you have a close, comfortable relationship in which neither of you is reluctant to speak out. Your attorney must be completely knowledgeable about the case, and you must be comfortable with his or her approach to your defense.

Settlement

Whether to settle will be an issue from the time an incident occurs through a final verdict, and perhaps beyond. Although settlement is not usually a formal part of pretrial or trial procedures, substantially more cases are settled rather than contested to a conclusion. You should be aware of what a settlement is, when it can be used, and what your rights are.

A settlement is an agreement made between parties to an incident, claim, or lawsuit that resolves their legal dispute. A settlement is often a financial disposition of a case without a decision on the merits. In most instances, payment is made to the plaintiff in exchange for a release, a legal document that absolves the defendant from all past, present, and future liability in connection with the incident. Most releases specifically state that the settlement by the defendant is not an admission of fault.

Any settlement that results in a payment on your behalf by an insurance company or anyone else other than yourself must be reported to the National Practitioner Data Bank. (See the "National Practitioner Data Bank" section for a discussion of the implications of having these data reported.)

There are substantial costs and risks involved in litigating a case to a conclusion. The longer a case lasts, the more time, effort, and money are expended.

SETTLEMENT PERSPECTIVES

Each of the participants in the litigation process has reasons for preferring settlement. The judge hearing the case wants to clear the court's calendar and dispose of cases quickly. To accomplish this, the judge may require the parties to participate in a pretrial settlement conference. Some states require that all cases go through alternate procedures before trial in an effort to settle. In some cases, the judge may actively serve as a settlement mediator.

The insurance carrier has a financial interest in the settlement of the case. A settlement would limit defense costs and establish a fixed sum for payment. By avoiding a trial, an uncertain jury verdict is eliminated.

A plaintiff's attorney considers a settlement a victory because it assures compensation to the client and compensation for the attorney's time and effort. By the same token, a plaintiff would favor a settlement because it assures compensation for damages and avoids further delay in receiving funds that may be needed for medical or rehabilitation purposes.

A defense attorney may consider a settlement in the case if a defense jury verdict is in doubt. A defendant physician may also accept a settlement rather than face the uncertainty of a trial. A settlement would also allow a defendant physician to avoid a potential verdict that may exceed his or her insurance coverage. Another reason a physician may wish to settle is to eliminate further commitment of time and energy to the litigation process.

SETTLEMENT FACTORS

During the course of any discussion regarding settlement, myriad factors come into play. Evidentiary concerns that would influence the decision to settle include unavailable witnesses and illegible, altered, or missing medical records. A settlement may be appropriate if there is a lack of expert witness support for the plaintiff or the defense or a questionable quality of expert opinion for the plaintiff or the defense.

Settlement discussions should include consideration of the amount of damages the plaintiff has sustained, the seriousness of the plaintiff's injuries, and the influence of the "sympathy factor" on a jury. The parties to the lawsuit may consider settlement if their case has been reviewed by a mandated pretrial screening panel. The panel's decision may be admissible in evidence at trial.

The dollar amount needed to reach a settlement agreement will be a big influence on whether a case is settled. The decision should take into consideration the verdict potential—either the estimated amount or the fact that the plaintiff's demand exceeds the limits of insurance coverage. If a personal defense counsel is retained to protect the defendant physician's assets, he or she will be interested in settling within the physician's policy limits.

Parties to the case will want to consider the jurisdiction in which the case will be tried. What are the previous jury verdicts in similar cases? What is the length of time needed to litigate the case to a conclusion?

Your defense team should consider your attitude. You may be adamant to go to trial or may not want to invest further time and energy in the case. Your attorneys will evaluate the adversarial position of the codefendants, if any. The parties should evaluate the strengths or weaknesses of individual witnesses, as well as the skill and reputation of the respective attorneys and the judge's reputation.

The possibility of a settlement may be discussed at any time. A case may be settled at the incident stage. This process is often referred to as *aggressive incident management*. The mechanics of this type of settlement differ from the mechanics of settlement of a formal claim.

SETTLEMENT OF AN INCIDENT

You will play a primary role in achieving a settlement at this stage. You should notify your insurance carrier early, as well as the hospital risk manager or incident manager if the incident occurred in the hospital. Whether a settlement offer is made to your patient depends on the response of the insurance carrier and/or the hospital. Further treatment of your patient at no cost may be suggested in exchange for a release. Some compensation to the patient may also be warranted.

SETTLEMENT OF A FORMAL CLAIM

Attorneys play a primary role in settling a case once a formal claim is filed. The plaintiff's attorney typically makes a monetary demand for settlement to the defense attorney. The defense attorney responds with denial, acceptance, or counteroffer. If a counteroffer is made, negotiations may continue until the parties arrive at an acceptable settlement figure. Demands or counteroffers can be made at any time even if settlement negotiations have previously broken down.

The insurance company also plays a critical role. The insurance company retains the authority to negotiate all settlements. The defense attorney can only accept a settlement demand or make a counteroffer with the consent of the insurance carrier.

Your rights regarding the settlement decision are contained in the policy. You may not have the right to accept or reject settlement; the insurance carrier and the defense attorney can agree to settle without your consent, but you may be consulted about your feelings on the matter. Defendants who do have that right will be consulted before any offers or counteroffers of settlement are made. You will be asked to sign a written consent to a proposed settlement.

You should review the terms of your insurance policy to determine whether you have the right to accept or reject a settlement. Whatever the case, you should be informed by your attorney of all settlement demands and counteroffers. You should be informed of the choices, the risks with each approach, and the alternatives that are available. Failure to keep you fully advised of settlement negotiations may constitute bad faith on the part of your insurance carrier, especially if the amount of a trial verdict exceeds your coverage. If the amount of the claim does exceed your policy limits, your personal defense attorney can play a significant role. He or she will serve as your intermediary to your insurance carrier and assigned defense counsel on settlement discussions and negotiations, will ensure that your rights are protected, and will pursue your remedies for a breach of those rights. (See "Professional Liability Insurance" for a discussion of when it is appropriate to retain personal defense counsel.)

You should take advantage of the expertise of your attorneys in the area of settlement. At the very least, you should be given an estimate of your chances of success at trial. To try an indefensible case that could have been settled would be a total waste of time and effort. On the other hand, to settle a defensible case may set a bad precedent and have adverse implications for your future practice and insurability. You should be as realistic and as objective as possible. Regardless of your decision, do not hesitate to make your feelings known to your defense attorney.

National Practitioner Data Bank

When you as a physician are involved in a lawsuit, you need to consider the implications of the National Practitioner Data Bank. Any payments, including settlements, made on your behalf by an insurance company or anyone other than yourself in a medical malpractice case are required to be reported to the Data Bank. Individual physicians are no longer required to report payments they make on their own behalf.

WHAT IS THE DATA BANK?

The National Practitioner Data Bank is an information clearinghouse that collects and releases information related to the professional competence and conduct of physicians, dentists, and some other health care practitioners. The Data Bank releases the following information: reports of medical malpractice payments, reports of adverse licensure actions, reports of certain negative professional review actions, and reports of Medicare and Medicaid sanctions. Currently, the information in the Data Bank is confidential, but there have been repeated efforts in Congress to make the information available to the general public. Entities that are permitted access to the information must maintain its confidentiality. Hospitals, managed health care organizations, and insurance companies are among the entities that can request reports from the Data Bank. Therefore, if you are reported to the Data Bank, it has the potential to adversely affect your future employability or insurability.

WHAT GETS REPORTED?

An entity that makes a full or partial payment for your benefit in settlement of a medical malpractice claim or satisfaction of a medical malpractice judgment against you must report the payment information to the Data Bank. Any payment made as a result of a suit or a claim solely against an entity (eg, a hospital, clinic, or group practice) that does not identify you, the individual practitioner, is not reportable.

Reportable medical malpractice payments are limited to the exchange of money and must be the result of a written Complaint or claim demanding monetary payment for damages. The written Complaint or claim must be based on allegations concerning your provision of, or failure to provide, health care services, and can include, but is not limited to, the filing of a cause of action based upon tort law.

Hospitals and other health care entities must report any professional review actions, based on your professional competence or conduct, that adversely affect your clinical privileges for more than 30 days. Such actions include reducing, restricting, suspending, revoking, or denying privileges, and also include an entity's decision not to renew your privileges, if that decision was based on your competence or conduct. In addition, hospitals and other health care entities must report the acceptance of your voluntary surrender or restriction of clinical privileges while you are under investigation for possible professional incompetence or improper professional conduct, or in return for not conducting an investigation or professional review action.

State medical licensing boards must report to the Data Bank certain disciplinary actions taken against your license related to professional competence or conduct. Professional societies also must report review actions related to professional competence or conduct that are taken through a formal peer review process and that adversely affect your membership.

If your lawsuit results in a report to the Data Bank, you will receive a notification that will include the report in its entirety. You should review the report for accuracy and follow the required procedures if you feel the report is factually incorrect or does not meet the reporting requirements. There are also Data Bank procedures that would allow you to add a statement of a limited number of characters to the report, with or without disputing the report. Once the Data Bank processes a statement or a dispute, it is sent to all entities that previously received that report and will be included with the report when it is disclosed in future requests.

Discovery

Discovery refers to pretrial procedures used by the parties to the lawsuit to gather and learn of evidence so as to develop their respective cases and to minimize the element of surprise at the time of the trial. These typically include Requests for Documents, Interrogatories, and Depositions but can also include Requests for Admission of Facts and Requests for Genuineness of Documents.

Discovery can eliminate unnecessary issues and enable the parties to either settle the case or present it for trial in an efficient manner. Through discovery procedures, attorneys can assess the strengths and weaknesses of both sides. Because depositions are the most important of the discovery procedures for a defendant physician, they will be discussed in a separate section.

INTERROGATORIES

Interrogatories are a set of written questions submitted by one party to the lawsuit to an opposing party, who must answer in writing under oath within a certain period of time. The answers are admissible at trial under certain circumstances. Interrogatories are more important than most people think. Therefore, your responses must be precise, thorough, and truthful.

Usually your defense attorney will draft the Answers to Interrogatories based on information that you have provided in pretrial consultations. You should carefully review with your attorney all of the Answers before they are signed and sworn to by you. You and your attorney will have to live with your responses throughout the litigation. Answers to Interrogatories may be used to cross-examine you at trial.

If you wish, you can offer to assist your attorney in preparing Interrogatories to be submitted to an opposing party. You might know critical information about the other party that should be brought out in this format.

REQUEST FOR ADMISSION OF FACTS

A Request for Admission of Facts is a series of factual statements, usually limited in number, served by one party to a lawsuit on another. The party served with the request is required to admit or deny the factual statements, in writing and under oath, within a prescribed period of time. Once a fact is admitted by an opposing party, that fact is no longer in controversy and can be introduced at trial without having to offer evidence to prove it.

A Request for Admission of Facts is an important discovery procedure that may be overlooked by many defense attorneys. For example, if you are a codefendant who was only marginally involved in the treatment of the plaintiff, a Request for Admission of Facts could provide the basis for a quick Motion for Summary Judgment in your favor. If you are the primary defendant, a Request for Admission of Facts can still simplify the disputed facts and shorten the ultimate trial. You should consult with your attorney regarding the advisability of using this discovery procedure and assist him or her in formulating the factual statements for the request.

REQUEST FOR ADMISSION OF GENUINENESS OF DOCUMENTS

A Request for Admission of Genuineness of Documents is a request from one party to a lawsuit to another. This request asks the opposing party to admit the authenticity of certain documents. In a medical malpractice lawsuit, the documents usually admitted by this procedure would be the medical records. If the plaintiff has had relevant prior or subsequent treatment from another physician or medical facility, this procedure can also be used to admit those records without the necessity of testimony from the other physician or the medical records librarian. This procedure is principally beneficial in simplifying both the trial itself and the procedures related to the introduction of documents at trial.

Depositions

Depositions are the most important discovery procedure. Every party to the lawsuit can examine the other party or any person who may possibly be a witness. This examination, officially recorded and taken under oath, is admissible at trial under certain circumstances. Your testimony at your deposition has great significance; you should not be fooled if it is taken in an informal setting or atmosphere. You should be just as prepared for your deposition as you would be for your trial testimony. The importance of a deposition cannot be overemphasized—remember that it may be introduced as evidence during the trial.

WHAT IS A DEPOSITION?

A deposition is a question-and-answer session in which the attorneys of the parties are present and involved in the examination and cross-examination of the witness. There are multiple purposes of a deposition. The primary purpose is to discover facts and supplement testimony and evidence obtained from other sources. Depositions are also used to obtain admissions from the opposing party, to lock in the testimony of a witness (especially one that may be unavailable at trial), to learn the identity of other possible witnesses, to learn the opposing expert's opinions and theories, to narrow facts and issues before trial, and to evaluate the case for settlement.

The procedure at a deposition is different from that which will take place at trial. The plaintiff's attorney will begin the questioning and will be allowed to cross-examine you and ask leading questions. Your defense attorney's role will be to object, when appropriate, and instruct you whether to answer the question. After the plaintiff's attorney has completed this questioning, your attorney probably will question you. Do not be surprised or disappointed, however, if you are not questioned by your attorney; in most instances, he or she is electing to preserve critical defense testimony until the time of trial.

HOW DO YOU PREPARE FOR YOUR DEPOSITION?

Preparation for your deposition is vital. Your testimony can be used to impeach your credibility if you offer contradictory testimony at trial. You should remember that what you say during your deposition is under oath. If you are not prepared, you may be trapped into saying something that you will later regret.

Before your deposition, you and your defense attorney should thoroughly discuss your knowledge of the facts of the case and the subjects on which you may be examined. It is important that you and your attorney devote sufficient time to this preparation.

As part of your preparation for your deposition, you will be instructed by your defense attorney to review the entire history of the case. You will need to familiarize yourself with all pertinent medical records, X-rays, test results, and data so that you can refer to this material easily. If you were asked to prepare a chronologic summary of the incident by your defense attorney, you should carefully review it before the deposition. It is often helpful to review the literature in any area of your specialty that may be the subject of questioning. You should have a complete understanding of the alternative treatment options that were available in the case and be prepared to explain the choice that you recommended to your patient.

Effective preparation for your deposition is not something that should be done at the last minute. If your deposition is approaching and you have not heard from your defense attorney, you should call your attorney and schedule a predeposition conference. Your defense attorney should set aside enough time to thoroughly prepare you for this event.

As part of the predeposition preparation, your attorney should question you and critique your answers. During this rehearsal your attorney should be able to identify the danger areas and weak points of your testimony and suggest alternative approaches.

In addition to explaining the process and setting of the deposition, your attorney should alert you to possible tactics of the plaintiff's attorney. In particular, you will be warned of repetitious or leading questions, which are calculated to put you on the defensive, wear you down, or irritate you. An attorney using the repetitious questions tactic may ask the same question over and over again, with slight changes in the wording. The purpose of this tactic is to make you angry or cause you to lose your temper or make a damaging admission. The attorney using the leading questions tactic is trying to get a yes or no response from you by beginning a question with "Wouldn't you agree, Doctor . . ." or "Is it not true . . . ." Think for yourself, and do not let the opposing attorney put words in your mouth. You do not have to answer these questions with a simple yes or no response.

Your defense attorney should warn you of the dangers of hypothetical questions. The opposing attorney may ask you to "assume" certain facts and express an opinion based on those facts. You may become trapped into being an expert witness for the plaintiff. Before answering, make sure that the "assumed" facts are consistent with this case and your opinion is consistent with your defense. Some plaintiff's attorneys will try to paint you into a corner. You should not boast when you are requested to acknowledge the breadth of your medical reading, because you may be held accountable for its content.

In addition, opposing counsel may try to get you to define an "absolute standard of care" in your case. Remember, at trial your admissions may be your downfall.

You should not allow yourself to be confused or appear to be confused by the proceedings. It might suggest that you were equally confused in treating the patient.

Finally, you should be careful about conceding medical authoritativeness. When asked if someone or a particular text is an authority, your attorney may want you to respond to the effect that "medicine is an art and not an exact science." Therefore, you do not always agree with everything written by any one author or found in any one particular text. You should ask the plaintiff's attorney to specify the particular section of the text or article, review its language, and carefully consider your position.

You should not be surprised if the plaintiff is present at your deposition. A party to a lawsuit has an absolute right to attend all depositions in person.

HOW SHOULD YOU CONDUCT YOURSELF AT YOUR DEPOSITION?

You must take the deposition seriously even if it is conducted in an informal atmosphere. If you have a strong case and perform well at the deposition, you may convince the plaintiff's side that they have no case. Most medical–legal commentators indicate that the strength of the defendant's testimony is one of the most critical factors in a case. Even if you do not perform well, the deposition is a good way to prepare you for what is ahead.

To be an effective witness, you should listen carefully to the questions, weigh your responses, and give yourself time to think before answering. It is always a good idea to take a short pause before answering a question; this gives your defense attorney a chance to object to the question if necessary. If your attorney objects to a question, do not answer it until you are instructed to do so.

If you do not understand a question, ask for it to be repeated and clarified before you respond. If you do not know an answer to a question, it is perfectly all right, indeed preferable, to say "I don't know." You should not be equivocal in your answers unless uncertainty is inherent in the medicine of the case. You should not ramble or volunteer information that goes beyond the scope of the question. You should not go off on a tangent defending yourself. Your defense attorney will give you that opportunity later in the deposition or at trial.

Although you may be upset by the deposition process, it is important to remain emotionally cool. It is almost always a mistake to argue with opposing counsel. This may be what the plaintiff's attorney is attempting to make you do, because an emotional outburst may be used to discredit you at trial. Although a deposition can be time-consuming, you should not show exasperation, boredom, or fatigue.

Because your deposition is being recorded, it is important to speak clearly and distinctly so that you can be understood. You should not act in a patronizing manner to the plaintiff's attorney, even if the questions are simplistic or inappropriate. Although the deposition process is often informal, you should dress neatly, be courteous, and take care in your manner, appearance, and remarks. Finally, you should keep in mind that the opposing attorneys in the case may be acquaintances or even friends. You should not be upset if there is friendly banter or conversation between them.

DEPOSITION OF ANOTHER

Because you are a party to the lawsuit, you have an absolute right to attend all of the depositions in person. This right is frequently disregarded, especially in view of the time constraints of a busy medical practice. It is extremely important to make every effort to be present at the depositions of the plaintiff and key opposing expert witnesses. Your presence could have an effect on the testimony given. Witnesses are more likely to tell the truth in your presence.

You should remember that testimony at a deposition is subject to all the responsibilities and penalties of testifying in court. In addition, attendance at the deposition of another is informative and can aid you in preparing for your own deposition or trial testimony. You may also be able to provide on-the-spot assistance to your attorney in his or her examination of the witness. Although there may be a significant amount of time and expense involved (such as travel out of state for the testimony of the plaintiff's expert), it is often worth your while in the long run. Plaintiff's experts, in particular, may be reluctant to be critical of your care in your presence. You should ask your defense attorney about your attendance at these depositions. In some cases, your insurance carrier may pay for your expenses to attend the deposition of the plaintiff's expert.

Trial

As your trial date approaches, you must clear your calendar. The trial should claim first priority on your time. In preparing for your trial, you should follow the steps you took in preparing for your deposition. It is vital that you become very familiar with the transcript of your deposition.

A large majority of medical malpractice cases are jury trials. Jury selection takes place immediately before the trial begins. Ask your defense attorney if he or she would like you to participate in this activity. You might make useful suggestions and can discuss your impressions with your counsel. This can be especially helpful if you practice in a small community and have personal knowledge of the people in the jury pool.

A typical jury trial consists of opening statements, the presentation of evidence (including witness testimony), closing arguments, instructions to the jury, verdict, and postverdict.

OPENING STATEMENTS

After the jury is selected, the opening statements are made by the attorneys for each of the parties to the lawsuit. The opening statements allow the attorneys to outline what they intend to prove or what the evidence will show. The attorneys are supposed to limit themselves to a factual outline and not engage in legal argument at this stage. This usually means that the attorneys cannot engage in theatrical statements as to why their client should prevail.

The plaintiff's attorney goes first, because the plaintiff has the burden of proof. Your attorney and the attorneys for your codefendants, if any, usually follow. In some cases, a defense attorney may choose to reserve his or her opening statement until the beginning of the defendant's case. If your case is not a jury trial, the opening statements will often be shortened or eliminated.

PRESENTATION OF EVIDENCE

The facts of the case are presented to the trier of fact—either a jury or a judge in a court trial—through various witnesses and exhibits. The plaintiff's goal during this phase of the trial is to produce facts that will convince the trier of fact that you were negligent and that your negligence directly caused injury to the plaintiff. The plaintiff has the burden of proving this by a preponderance of the evidence, which simply means more likely true than not true, or 51% likely. If the plaintiff has alleged that you committed gross negligence, a higher burden of proof of clear and convincing evidence is imposed on that portion of the claim.

The plaintiff attempts to meet the burden by introducing evidence through witnesses, medical documents, exhibits, etc. The most critical evidence for the plaintiff usually comes from one or more expert witnesses, who must testify that your care of the plaintiff did not meet the standard of care and that the failure to meet the standard caused injury to the plaintiff.

At the completion of the plaintiff's case, the defense will usually make a motion for a directed verdict. A directed verdict is a ruling by the trial judge that, as a matter of law, the verdict must be in favor of a particular party, usually because of a clear failure to meet the burden of proof. If the judge feels that the plaintiff has not introduced enough evidence to demonstrate that the basic elements of medical malpractice might have occurred, he or she will grant a directed verdict. Although it is rare for a trial judge to grant a directed verdict at this stage of a case, if it is granted, the case ends.

If the defense motion for a directed verdict is denied, it is your responsibility and that of your codefendants, if any, to present evidence in support of your defense. The defense goal is to either prove that there was no negligence whatsoever or that the plaintiff's injuries were not the direct result of your negligence. Like the plaintiff, the defense side attempts to meet this goal by introducing evidence through medical documents, witnesses, exhibits, etc. Expert witnesses for the defense are also critical in establishing that the standard of care was met, or that the plaintiff's injuries were not the result of a deviation from the standard of care. Demonstrative evidence, such as charts, anatomic models, and videotapes, can be helpful in educating the jury and/or the trial judge about the medicine involved in the case.

Upon completion of the defense case, the plaintiff is entitled to offer rebuttal evidence. This evidence is usually limited to new evidence that was introduced during the presentation of the defense case. The plaintiff is given the right of rebuttal under our system of law because the burden of proof is on the plaintiff.

WITNESS TESTIMONY

Although many types of evidence can be introduced during the plaintiff's and defendant's case, the direct testimony of witnesses is among the most important, especially in jury trials. This testimony is elicited by direct examination and cross-examination.

Direct examination is the questioning of a witness by the attorney who has called that witness to the stand. During direct examination, the attorney may not ask leading questions, unless the witness is considered a "hostile witness." If the trial judge determines that a witness is "hostile"—in other words, may favor the opposing side to the litigation—the attorney who called the witness is permitted to treat the questioning as a cross-examination (see below) and can ask leading questions. If you are called as a witness by the plaintiff's attorney, you will likely be declared a hostile witness.

Cross-examination is the subsequent questioning by an opposing attorney of a witness who is already on the witness stand. The attorney is allowed to ask leading questions during cross-examination.

CLOSING ARGUMENTS

The attorneys' final arguments to the jury are presented in the closing arguments. In a court trial, closing arguments are still presented to the trial judge, but they are usually shorter and more legalistic.

Closing arguments allow the attorneys to summarize their cases and argue why their clients should prevail. The plaintiff's attorney goes first, followed by the defense attorney (or attorneys, if there are codefendants in the case). The plaintiff's attorney is given a final opportunity to make a rebuttal argument after the defense attorneys have finished.

After the completion of the presentation of the evidence, the defense usually renews a motion for a directed verdict. In a large majority of cases this motion is denied, and the jury is allowed to deliberate and reach a verdict.

INSTRUCTIONS TO THE JURY

Before a case is formally given to a jury for deliberation, the judge instructs the jurors on the applicable law for the case. The judge explains the legal principles and provides guidelines that govern the jury deliberations. The judge will discuss damages, but will also instruct the jurors not to consider damages unless the jury finds in favor of the plaintiff on the issue of malpractice.

Instructions to the jury are obviously not required in a case that is tried by a judge without a jury.

VERDICT

After completing deliberations, the jury (or the judge in a court trial) renders a formal decision in the case, which is known as the verdict. The verdict must be in favor of either the plaintiff or the defendant. In the case of multiple defendants, there can be a split verdict that finds in favor of some, but not all, of the defendants. Damages must be awarded to the plaintiff when the verdict is in favor of the plaintiff, even if the damages are in a small amount (known as *nominal damages*). There are no damages awarded in the case of a complete defense verdict.

POSTVERDICT

A medical malpractice case does not necessarily end when a verdict is rendered. All of the parties to the lawsuit have a number of options if the verdict is unfavorable. If a verdict has been entered against you as a defendant, your attorneys can ask the trial court to set aside the verdict and grant a new trial; ask the trial court to change the verdict by entering a judgment in your favor; ask the trial court to reduce the amount of the damage award (known as *remittitur*); reopen settlement negotiations with the plaintiff, using the threat of appeal as leverage; or file an appeal.

If the verdict was in your favor, in other words, a defense verdict, the plaintiff has a similar range of options. The plaintiff's attorneys can ask the trial court to set aside the verdict and grant a new trial; ask the trial court to change the verdict by entering a judgment in favor of the plaintiff; reopen settlement negotiations, using the threat of appeal as leverage; or file an appeal. In some jurisdictions, a plaintiff who won the case can ask the trial judge to increase the amount of damages awarded, a process which is known as *additur*.

How to Be an Effective Witness at Trial

Preparation is vital to your trial testimony. As a start, review the above "Depositions" section. All of the points made there are equally applicable to your trial testimony. In this section, we will focus on those items that pertain specifically to the trial.

Your testimony at trial may be the single most important factor in determining whether you will win or lose your case. Your presence during the entire trial is important, because it conveys your concern to the judge and jury. In addition to the facts of the case, a judge or jury is likely to take into consideration your appearance, professionalism, and manner.

PRETRIAL PREPARATION

You should review the transcript of your deposition testimony and the transcripts of the experts' depositions, especially if the depositions took place a long time ago. You need to understand the strengths and weaknesses of your case before the trial begins.

You will also need to spend a substantial amount of time with your attorney preparing for trial. You should insist on a timely pretrial conference with your attorney if your attorney has not scheduled one and the trial is approaching.

Often it is helpful for you to have your family, friends, and even selected members of your staff present during the trial. Their presence will give you moral support in this stressful time. It will also make an impression on the jury.

TRIAL TESTIMONY

If you and your attorney decide that it is in your best interest for you to testify on your own behalf, you should take the time now to consider how to conduct yourself on the stand. Most important, you should tell the truth. If two of your responses are inconsistent, do not collapse, because your attorney can give you an opportunity to explain. There is no reason to panic if you are caught in a mistake.

You must understand the question before you attempt to answer it. You cannot give an accurate answer unless you understand the question. If you need to, you can ask the attorney to repeat the question. Also, you need to be cautious in responding to leading or repetitive questions. When you give an answer, you do not have to volunteer more information than the question calls for. You also do not have to accept the opposing counsel's summary of your testimony unless it is accurate.

It is best to speak directly to the jury and not talk down to them. You should not be afraid to look the jury members in the eye and speak to them as frankly and openly as you would to a friend or neighbor. You don't want to look at your lawyer for help when you are on the stand. The jury would notice this and get a bad impression.

The judge may ask you a question, so do not be surprised. You should answer it unless your attorney objects.

You need to be articulate—speak clearly and audibly. You should try to avoid mannerisms of speech, such as mumbling or speaking rapidly and using "umms" and "you knows."

Being respectful and courteous at all times is a good way to make a favorable impression on the court and jury. You should be sure to answer politely and to address the judge as "Your Honor." Do not be smug or project an attitude of "I know it all."

No matter how hard you are pressed, you should not lose your temper. You should not argue with the attorney on the other side. Remember, the plaintiff's attorney has the right to question you.

Hidden Messages in Body Language

- Slouching may indicate a sloppy practice.
- Placing your hand over your mouth when you speak could suggest that you have something to hide.
- Folded arms may be considered a defensive gesture.

Habits to Avoid

- Scowling
- Fidgeting on the witness stand
- Tugging at your ear
- Wringing your hands
- Biting your fingernails

The way you dress for your trial is important. Flashy dress may convey that you are more interested in making money than in taking care of patients. Untidy appearance may indicate that you are disorganized and unreliable.

You need to be aware of your body language because you may be sending the wrong message to the jury. Also, you should be aware of nonverbal communication or distracting habits. The potential for sending inaccurate signals to the jury is high.

Finally, rather than manifesting relief, triumph, or defeat when you leave the witness stand, you should walk with confidence at a normal pace.

Appendix

COMMONSENSE GLOSSARY OF MEDICAL-LEGAL TERMS

Abandonment: Termination of a physician–patient relationship without reasonable notice and without an opportunity for the patient to acquire adequate medical care, which results in some type of damage to the patient.

Additur: The power of the trial court to assess damages or increase the amount of an inadequate award; it cannot be done without the defendant's consent. Also, it is not permitted in tort claims within the federal system.

Admissibility (in evidence): Evidence that may be introduced properly in a legal proceeding. The determination of admissibility is based on legal rules of evidence and is made by the trial judge or a screening panel.

Admissions: Voluntary acknowledgments of the existence of certain facts by a party to a legal proceeding. In a malpractice proceeding, an admission typically would be a statement of culpability by a defendant.

Affidavit: A voluntary, written statement of facts made under oath before an officer of the court or before a notary public.

Affirmative defense: A defendant's response to a claim that challenges the plaintiff's legal right to bring the claim. The defendant must raise the defense and has the burden of proof. The truth of the claim is not contested; examples are statute of limitations, assumption of risk, and contributory negligence.

Allegation: A statement of a party to an action, made in a pleading, setting out what the party expects to prove.

Answer: A defendant's written response to a complaint or declaration in a legal proceeding. The answer typically either denies the allegations of the plaintiff or makes new allegations as to why the plaintiff should not recover damages.

Appeal: The process by which a decision of a lower court is brought for review to a court of higher jurisdiction, seeking a reversal or a new trial.

Appellant: The party who brings an appeal of one court's decision to another court or jurisdiction.

Appellate court: The court that reviews trial court decisions. Appellate courts review the transcript of the trial court proceedings and determine whether there were errors of law committed by the trial court.

Appellee: The opposing party in an appeal; sometimes referred to as the respondent.

Arbitration: A method of dispute resolution in which a neutral third party (arbitrator) renders a decision after a hearing at which both parties are given the opportunity to present their cases. The decision can be binding or nonbinding depending upon state law and/or the prior agreement of the parties.

Attorney work product: Materials used by an attorney in preparation for litigation. These materials usually are not subject to discovery.

Bailiff: An officer of the court who is in charge of courtroom decorum and who directs witnesses to the witness stand and attends to the jurors.

Battery: The unauthorized and offensive touching of a person by another. In medical malpractice cases, battery is typically contact of some type with a patient who has not consented to the contact. Battery can be either a civil or a criminal offense.

Bench trial: A trial without a jury, wherein the judge determines the facts as well as the law. Also known as a court trial.

Burden of proof: The legal responsibility or duty of affirmatively proving a fact or facts in a dispute. The plaintiff typically has the burden of proof.

Captain of the ship: A doctrine whereby the surgeon in charge of a medical team is liable for all the negligent acts of the members of the team.

Captive insurance company: A company owned and controlled by those it insures, such as a hospital, hospital association, medical society, or medical specialty society establishing its own medical malpractice insurance company.

Case: An action or cause of action; a matter in dispute; a lawsuit.

Case law: Legal principles derived from judicial decisions. Case law differs from statutory law, which is enacted by legislatures. Case law is also known as common law.

Cause of action: A set of alleged facts that a plaintiff uses to seek legal redress.

Claims-made insurance policy: A policy that covers only those claims submitted during the term of the policy. Insurance coverage ceases on the date the policy is terminated unless reporting endorsement (tail coverage) is purchased. It is desirable that a claims-made policy include a guarantee for purchase of reporting endorsement coverage and waiver of premium for reporting endorsement coverage in the event of death, disability, or retirement (insurance companies' definitions of retirement may vary).

Clear and convincing proof: A higher degree of proof than required in the ordinary civil action (preponderance of evidence) but less than the degree required in a criminal case (beyond a reasonable doubt).

Clerk of the court: The person who is responsible for the administrative functions of the court. During a trial, the clerk administers the oaths to the witnesses, receives and marks exhibits into evidence, and requests the verdict from the jurors.

Collateral source: A rule of law that prevents a court from subtracting from the damage award any payments that the plaintiff has received from such sources as workers' compensation, health insurance, government benefits, or sick pay benefits.

Commercial insurance company: A for-profit company owned and controlled by stockholders (stock company) or policyholders (mutual company).

Common law: That body of law that was passed down to the colonies by the British legal system and has been interpreted and refined by case law, as opposed to statutory law. It is also known as case law.

Comparative negligence: Most states have adopted this affirmative defense that compares the negligence of the defendant to that of the plaintiff. The plaintiff may recover damages from a negligent defendant even if the plaintiff and defendant are equally at fault. However, the plaintiff's damages are reduced in proportion to his or her own fault. It is only when the plaintiff's negligence is greater than the defendant's that there can be no recovery.

Complaint: A legal document that is the initial pleading on the part of the plaintiff in a civil lawsuit. This document states the alleged facts and bases of the cause(s) of action and requests damages or other relief. The Complaint is usually attached to the Summons. A Complaint is sometimes known as a Declaration.

Contingency fee: A fee agreement between the plaintiff and the plaintiff's attorney, whereby the plaintiff agrees to pay the attorney a percentage of the damages recovered.

Contributory negligence: An affirmative defense that prevents any recovery or award of damages against a defendant when the plaintiff's own negligence contributed to his or her own injury in any degree, even though the defendant's negligence also may have contributed to the injury.

Counterclaim: A separate cause of action brought by a defendant against the plaintiff in opposition or as an offset to the claim of the plaintiff. A counterclaim must be brought in the same legal proceeding filed by the plaintiff and must relate to the subject matter of the litigation.

Court reporter: A professionally trained stenographer who transcribes deposition or trial testimony.

Court trial: A trial without a jury, wherein the judge determines the facts as well as the law. Also known as a bench trial.

Cross-claim: A separate cause of action brought by a party to a lawsuit against another party on the same side. Cross-claims typically are brought by one defendant against another.

Culpability: Being at fault; deserving reproach or punishment for some act or course of action. Culpability connotes wrongdoing or errors of ignorance, omission, or negligence.

Damages: The sum of money a court or jury awards as compensation for a tort or breach of contract. The law recognizes certain categories of damages. These categories often are imprecise and inconsistent. Variations exist among jurisdictions, and all are not strictly adhered to by the courts. Damages either may be compensatory or punitive, depending on whether they are awarded as the measure of actual loss suffered or as punishment for outrageous conduct to deter future transgressions.

Defamation: An intentional false communication, either published or publicly spoken, which injures a person's reputation or good name; this includes both libel and slander. Statements made in a court proceeding cannot be the basis for a defamation claim.

Default judgment: A judgment entered against the defendant for the defendant's failure to answer the plaintiff's cause of action or to comply with any other required step in litigation, including failure to appear and put on a defense at trial.

Defendant: The party against whom relief is sought in an action; in a criminal case, the accused.

Deposition: A pretrial discovery device by which one party to the action, typically through his or her attorney, asks oral questions of the other party, a witness for the other party, or any potential witness. The deposition is conducted under oath outside of the courtroom, usually in one of the attorneys' offices. A transcript is made of the deposition and is admissible at trial under certain circumstances.

Directed verdict: Ruling by the trial judge that, as a matter of law, the verdict must be in favor of a particular party. A verdict is usually directed as a result of a clear failure to meet the burden of proof, sometimes referred to as a failure to establish a prima facie case.

Discovery: Pretrial procedures used by the parties to the action to gather and learn of evidence in order to develop their respective cases and to minimize the element of surprise at the time of the trial. These typically include Requests for Documents, Interrogatories, and Depositions but also can include Requests for Admission of Facts and Requests for Genuineness of Documents.

Dismissal: An order or judgment finally disposing of an action, suit, motion, etc, without a trial on the issues. To dismiss a motion is to deny it; to dismiss an appeal is to affirm the judgment of the trial court.

Due process: Legal procedures that have been established in systems of jurisprudence for the enforcement and protection of private rights. It often means simply a fair trial or hearing.

Duty: An obligation recognized by the law. A physician's duty to a patient is to provide the degree of care ordinarily exercised by physicians practicing in the same community (local standard of care) or area of specialization (national standard of care).

Emancipated minor: A child less than 18 years of age who has the rights and duties of an adult and whose parent no longer has any rights and duties to the child. A minor can become emancipated by certain acts, such as becoming self-supporting, marrying, becoming a parent, or obtaining a court order. State laws vary a great deal on this issue.

Evidence: Facts presented at trial through witnesses, records, documents, concrete objects, etc., for the purpose of proving or defending a case.

Exclusions: Insurance policy provisions that specify the situations, procedures, occurrences, or persons not covered by the policy. Professional liability policies contain the usual insurance exclusions, such as for discrimination and contractually assumed liability; however, they also typically include provisions that exclude coverage for dishonest, fraudulent, or criminal acts, and punitive damages and intentional torts. Policies sometimes have exclusions for the liability of employees, sexual relations with patients, and injuries sustained from automobile accidents.

Expert opinion: The testimony of a person who has special training, knowledge, skill, or experience in an area relevant to resolution of the legal dispute and whose qualifications meet with the court's satisfaction. Expert witnesses are authorized to testify and render opinions based on their qualifications, rather than on personal knowledge of the facts in issue.

Federal court: Federal courts are a system of trial and appellate courts like state courts, which are limited in their power to hear cases. Medical malpractice cases generally are not filed in the federal courts unless the parties to the case are from different states or the case falls under the Federal Tort Claims Act. Federal courts include district courts, courts of appeals, and the Supreme Court.

Fiduciary: Having a special relationship toward another that imposes legal duties to act responsibly and in good faith to protect that party's interests.

Fraud: Intentional misrepresentation, concealment, or nondisclosure of a material fact that results in the injury of another.

Garnishment: The process by which a court orders money or goods controlled by a third person and owed or belonging to a defendant to be used to pay a plaintiff's award against the defendant.

Hearsay: An out-of-court statement offered in court to prove the truth of the facts contained in the statement. Hearsay is generally not admissible because there is usually no adequate basis for determining whether the out-of-court statement is true. There are, however, exceptions to the hearsay rule.

Hostile witness: A witness whose position or viewpoint is adverse to that of the party who called him or her to the stand.

Hung jury: A jury that cannot come to a decision that constitutes a verdict in its jurisdiction, frequently after lengthy deliberation. A hung jury results in a mistrial, which in most circumstances means the case will be retried before a new jury.

Hypothetical question: A question that solicits the opinion of an expert witness at a trial or deposition based on a combination of assumptions and facts already introduced in evidence.

Impeachment (of a witness): The process by which the truth or credibility of the testimony of a witness is challenged.

Impleader: The process by which a party to a lawsuit brings a new party into the lawsuit, alleging that the new party is responsible for all or part of the claim.

Incompetency: Lack of ability, knowledge, legal qualification, or fitness to perform a required duty or exercise a right. With respect to physicians, this typically refers to the inability or lack of fitness to practice medicine. With respect to patients, this usually refers to the inability to consent to a treatment or procedure.

Informed consent: The legal requirement that a patient be made aware of the nature and risks of a medical procedure or treatment before agreeing to its performance.

Injunction: A court order prohibiting a party to do or continue to do a particular act.

Insurance insolvency fund (guaranty fund): A state-administered fund that provides insurance coverage for policyholders of state-registered insurance entities that have gone out of business or become insolvent or bankrupt. This fund will not necessarily provide the same amount of coverage as provided in the original policy.

Interrogatories: A discovery procedure in which one party submits a series of written questions to the opposing party, who must answer in writing under oath within a certain period of time. The Answers are admissible at trial under certain circumstances.

Joint and several liability: A legal doctrine applied in negligence cases against multiple defendants in some jurisdictions. The injured party is entitled to recover the entire amount of damages awarded from a single defendant, irrespective of the percentage of negligence or responsibility of that defendant.

Joint Underwriting Association (JUA): A state-sponsored insurance company that has been created to make insurance available in tight market conditions. A JUA may or may not be required to provide professional liability insurance to all licensed physicians in the state, depending on state law. The solvency of the JUA is typically supported by assessments on insurance carriers licensed to do business in the state.

Judgment: The final determination of the rights of the parties to a suit that is binding unless it is overturned or modified on appeal.

Jury trial: A trial in which 12 or fewer individuals are summoned and sworn in to hear the evidence, determine the facts, and render a verdict.

Liability limits: The maximum sum or sums that an insurance company is obligated to pay for a settlement or judgment against an insured party. In medical professional liability policies, these limits are generally written with a limit per claim and a limit of aggregate liability for each year of coverage or policy period.

Libel: A false and malicious publication that injures the reputation of another.

Loss of consortium: A claim for damages by the spouse of an injured party for the loss of care, comfort, society, and sexual relations; often a part of an award of damages in a tort action for injury or wrongful death of a spouse.

Malpractice: Negligence by a professional. In medical terms, it is the failure to exercise that degree of care used by reasonably careful physicians of like qualifications in the same or similar circumstances. The patient's injury must be a result of this failure to meet this duty of care.

Motion: A written or oral request of the court to make an order or ruling in favor of the requesting party.

Negligence: Legal cause of action involving the failure to exercise the degree of diligence and care that a reasonably and ordinarily prudent person would exercise under the same or similar circumstances.

Occurrence insurance policy: An insurance policy that obligates the insurer to pay for claims that took place during the period covered by the policy, regardless of when the claim is filed. This type of policy does not require that the policyholder purchase reporting endorsement (tail) coverage upon termination.

Periodic payments: Damages paid to a plaintiff in installments instead of in one lump sum. If a state law permits it, periodic payments may be ordered when the damages exceed a certain amount.

Physician-owned insurance company: A company typically owned and controlled by physicians, but not required to be a nonprofit corporation. It might be a captive insurance company or a mutual insurance company.

Plaintiff: The party that files a lawsuit.

Pleadings: Legal documents filed in a lawsuit in which the issues in dispute are identified and clarified, including the plaintiff's cause of action and the defendant's grounds of defense. These documents typically are filed in the first phase of a lawsuit.

Precedent: A rule of law established for the first time by a court for a particular type of case and thereafter referred to in deciding similar cases subject to that court's jurisdiction.

Preponderance of evidence: The greater weight of evidence, or evidence that is more credible or convincing to the mind, leading the trier of fact to find the disputed issue exists more likely than not (ie, more than 50% likely). This is typically the standard of proof in civil cases not involving punitive damages.

Prior acts endorsement (nose coverage): A policy that backdates covered claims to a date before the inception of a policy. In some instances, this policy may be purchased from a new professional liability insurance carrier as an alternative to reporting endorsement (tail coverage).

Proximate cause: An act or omission that, in a natural and continuous sequence unbroken by any intervening cause, produces an injury. In a medical malpractice case, failure to adhere to the standard of care must be the proximate cause of the injury to the patient.

Rebut: Refute; present opposing evidence or arguments.

Reinsurance: Insurance purchased by a primary insurance carrier to reimburse it for settlements and judgments in excess of a specified limit.

Remittitur: The procedural process by which an excessive monetary verdict of the jury is reduced; it cannot be granted without a new trial unless the unfavored party consents.

Reporting endorsement (tail coverage): A special policy that extends the time for reporting claims under claims-made insurance, which is purchased from your existing carrier upon termination or cancellation of your policy. It is also typically provided by your current insurance carrier upon death, disability, or retirement. This type of coverage essentially converts a claims-made policy into an occurrence policy.

Reservation of rights: An insurance term that refers to a situation arising when your insurance carrier questions whether there is coverage for an incident of malpractice.

Res ipsa loquitur: "The thing speaks for itself." The legal theory in which it must be proven that the cause of the injury was in the defendant's exclusive control and that the accident was one that ordinarily does not happen in the absence of negligence. In medical malpractice cases, it allows a patient to prove his or her case without the necessity of an expert witness to testify that the defendant physician violated the standards of care. It is applicable only in those instances in which negligence is clear and obvious even to a layperson, such as foreign object cases in which a surgeon leaves a sponge in the patient following surgery.

Respondeat superior: "Let the master answer." The legal principle that makes an employer liable for civil wrongs committed by employees within the course and scope of their employment. In medical malpractice cases, this theory often is used to hold hospitals liable for the negligence of employees and attending physicians responsible for residents.

Risk-retention group: A special insurance entity that is limited to individuals or organizations engaged in similar activities with similar or related liability exposures; members must share a common business, trade, or profession. A risk-retention group is only required to comply with state insurance laws in its state of incorporation. Once a risk-retention group is licensed, it can then offer insurance in other states.

Self-insurance: The financial arrangements made by individuals and institutions that cannot, or choose not to, obtain commercial insurance to protect themselves against some or all of the risks arising out of their practice. These arrangements range from "going bare" (ie, having no insurance) to sophisticated multihospital programs that offer malpractice coverage to medical staff physicians.

Settlement: An agreement made between the parties to a lawsuit or a claim that resolves their legal dispute.

Slander: The speaking of false and malicious words that damage the reputation of another.

Standard of care: A measure of behavior upon which the legal theory of negligence is based. A physician is required to adhere to the standards of practice of reasonably competent physicians, in the same or similar circumstances, with comparable training and experience either in their own locality (local standard of care) or their own medical specialty (national standard of care).

Statute of limitations: The time period in which a plaintiff may file a lawsuit. Once this period expires, the plaintiff's lawsuit is barred if the defendant asserts the affirmative defense of the statute of limitations.

Statutory law: Laws enacted by a legislature.

Stipulation: An agreement made by both parties to the litigation regulating any matter related to the case, proceeding, or trial. For instance, litigants can agree to extend the time period for pleadings or to admit certain facts into evidence at trial. It is only binding if it is in writing, unless it was made on the record during the proceeding. It may require court approval.

Structured settlement: Settlement agreement between the parties to a lawsuit or a claim in which the damages are paid to the plaintiff over time instead of in one lump sum. These settlements usually are financed through the purchase of an annuity.

Subpoena: Court order requiring a witness to appear at a certain proceeding to give testimony and/or produce documents.

Summary judgment: Granting of a judgment in favor of either party before trial. Summary judgment is granted only when there is no factual dispute and one of the parties is entitled to judgment as a matter of law.

Summons: A legal document attached to the Complaint or Declaration in a lawsuit that notifies the defendant that he or she is being sued. It orders the defendant or the defendant's attorney to file a response within a specified period of time.

Tort: A civil wrong for which an action can be filed in court to recover damages for personal injury or property damage resulting from negligent acts or intentional misconduct.

Trier of fact: The jury or, in the case of trial without jury, the judge.

Underwriting: The selection process by which an insurance company evaluates the risk of loss and determines which of the risks (applicants) should be accepted. On an individual basis, underwriting would also determine the amounts and limits of coverage for individual applicants.

Verdict: The formal decision or finding made by a jury or judge. The verdict is in favor of the plaintiff or defendant, and damages are usually awarded when the verdict is in favor of the plaintiff.

Vicarious liability: Civil liability for the actions of others. Physicians may be vicariously liable for the negligent acts of their employees committed within the scope of their employment (*respondeat superior*). In the hospital setting, a surgeon may be vicariously liable for the negligent acts of all members of the surgical team (captain of the ship).

Wrongful birth: An action brought by parents who seek damages after the birth of an impaired child, in which the parents allege that negligent treatment or advice deprived them of the opportunity to avoid conception or terminate the pregnancy.

Wrongful conception/wrongful pregnancy: An action brought by parents who seek damages arising from a negligent performance of a sterilization procedure of abortion.

Wrongful life: An action brought by a child born with impairments who contends that he or she would not have been born but for negligent advice to, or treatment of, the parents.

CROSS-REFERENCE INDEX OF MEDICAL–LEGAL TERMS

Professional Liability Insurance

Captive insurance company
Claims-made insurance policy
Commercial insurance policy
Exclusions
Insurance insolvency fund
Joint Underwriting Association
Liability limits
Occurrence insurance policy
Physician-owned insurance company
Prior acts endorsement
Reinsurance
Reporting endorsement
Reservation of rights
Risk-retention group
Self-insurance
Underwriting

Incident Management

Abandonment
Battery
Culpability
Duty
Emancipated minor
Fiduciary
Fraud
Incompetency
Informed consent
Negligence

Claims Management

Affirmative defense
Allegation
Answer
Captain of the ship
Case
Cause of action
Comparative negligence
Complaint
Contributory negligence
Counterclaim
Cross-claim
Culpability

Damages
Defendant
Impleader
Interrogatories
Joint and several liability
Loss of consortium
Malpractice
Motion
Plaintiff
Pleadings
Proximate cause
Standard of care
Statute of limitations
Tort
Vicarious liability
Wrongful birth
Wrongful conception/wrongful
    pregnancy
Wrongful life

Settlement

Arbitration
Structured settlement

Discovery

Admissions
Affidavit
Attorney work product
Default judgment
Deposition
Subpoena
Summons

Trial

Additur
Admissibility
Appeal
Appellant
Appellate court
Appellee
Bailiff
Bench trial
Burden of proof

Case law	Hypothetical question
Clear and convincing proof	Impeachment
Clerk of the court	Injunction
Collateral source	Judgment
Common law	Jury trial
Contingency fee	Libel
Court reporter	Periodic payments
Court trial	Precedent
Defamation	Preponderance of evidence
Directed verdict	Rebut
Dismissal	Remittitur
Due process	*Res ipsa loquitur*
Evidence	*Respondeat superior*
Expert opinion	Slander
Federal court	Statutory law
Garnishment	Stipulation
Hearsay	Summary judgment
Hostile witness	Trier of fact
Hung jury	Verdict

SUGGESTED READING

If you are interested in reading about the subjects covered in the *Litigation Assistant* in more depth, the following publications are recommended.

Belli MM Sr, Carlova J. Belli for your malpractice defense. Oradell, New Jersey: Medical Economics Books, 1986

Charles SC, Kennedy E. Defendant: a psychiatrist on trial for medical malpractice. New York: The Free Press, 1985

Freedman MA. Society to L & D . . . stat! Saint Simons Island, Georgia: Marshwinds Advisory Company, 1988

Huber PW. Liability: the legal revolution and its consequences. New York: Basic Books, 1988

O'Connell J, Kelly CB. The blame game: injuries, insurance and injustice. Lexington, Massachusetts: DC Heath and Co, 1987

Olson WK. The litigation explosion: what happened when America unleashed the lawsuit. New York: Truman Talley Books–Dutton, 1991

Werth B. Damages. New York: Simon & Schuster, 1988